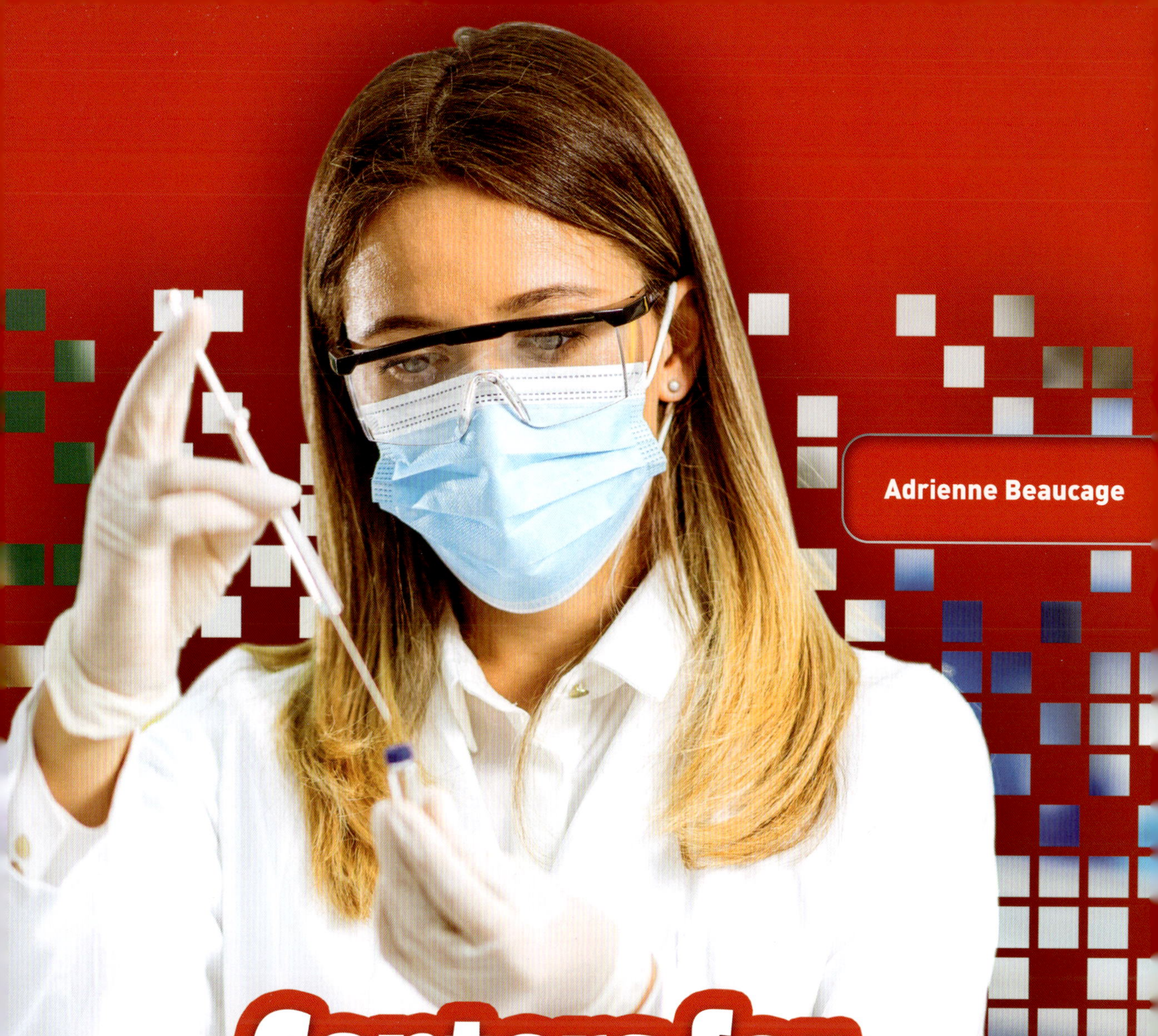

Adrienne Beaucage

Centers for Disease Control and Prevention

POWER • AUTHORITY • GOVERNANCE

LIGHTBOX
openlightbox.com

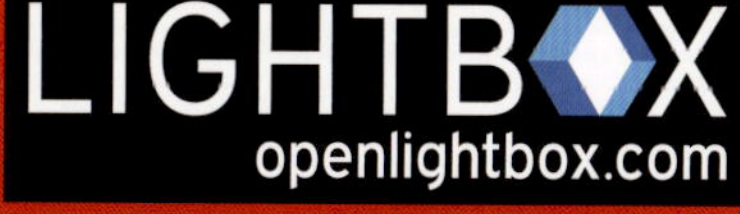

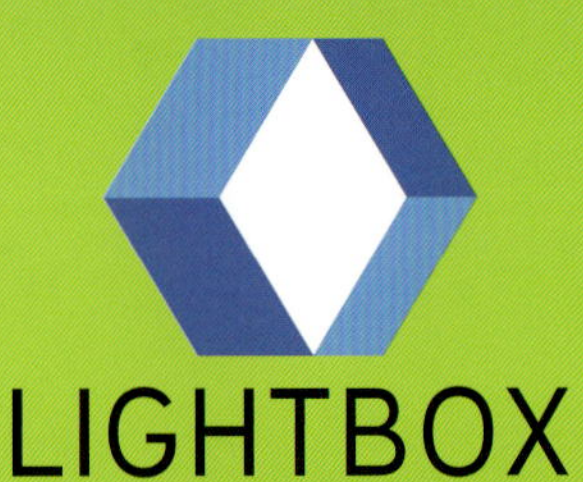

Go to
www.openlightbox.com
and enter this book's
unique code.

ACCESS CODE

LBXZ7837

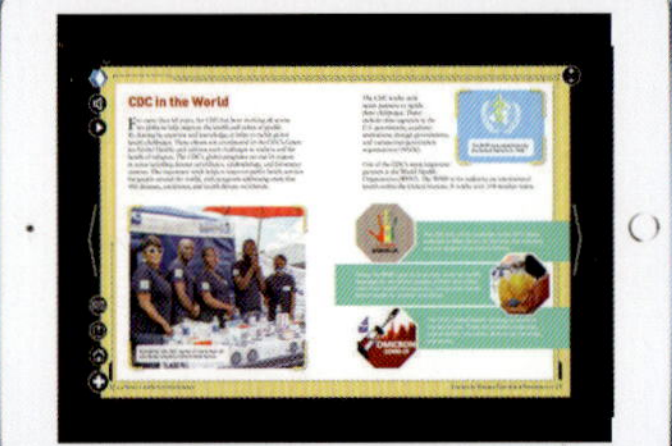

Lightbox is an all-inclusive digital solution for the teaching and learning of curriculum topics in an original, groundbreaking way. Lightbox is based on National Curriculum Standards.

LIGHTBOX SUPPLEMENTARY RESOURCES

SHARE
Share titles within your Learning Management System (LMS) or Library Circulation System

CURRICULUM
Find national and state curriculum correlations

CITATION
Create bibliographical references following APA, CMOS, and MLA styles

STANDARD FEATURES OF LIGHTBOX

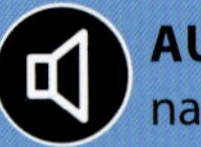

AUDIO High-quality narration using text-to-speech system

ACTIVITIES Printable PDFs that can be emailed and graded

SLIDESHOWS Pictorial overviews of key concepts

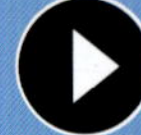

VIDEOS Embedded high-definition video clips

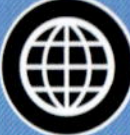

WEBLINKS Curated links to external, child-safe resources

TRANSPARENCIES Step-by-step layering of maps, diagrams, charts, and timelines

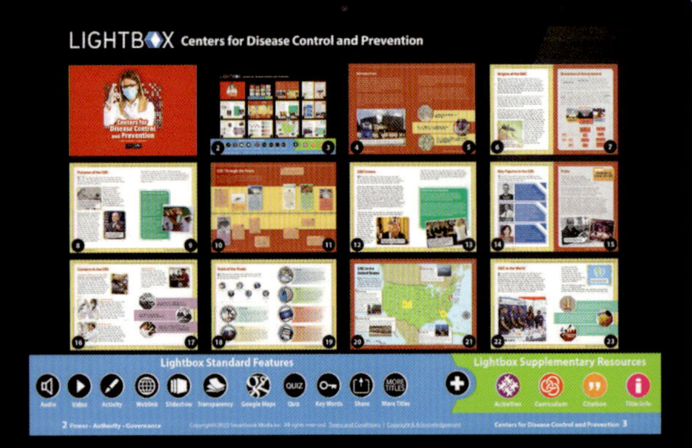

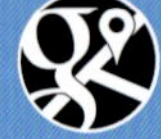

INTERACTIVE MAPS Interactive maps and aerial satellite imagery

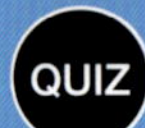

QUIZZES Ten multiple-choice questions that are automatically graded and emailed for teacher assessment

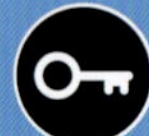

KEY WORDS Matching key concepts to their definitions

This title is part of our Lightbox digital subscription

Lightbox Grades 3–5 Subscription
ISBN 978-1-5105-5424-5

Access hundreds of Lightbox titles with our digital subscription. Sign up for a **FREE** subscription trial at **www.openlightbox.com/trial**

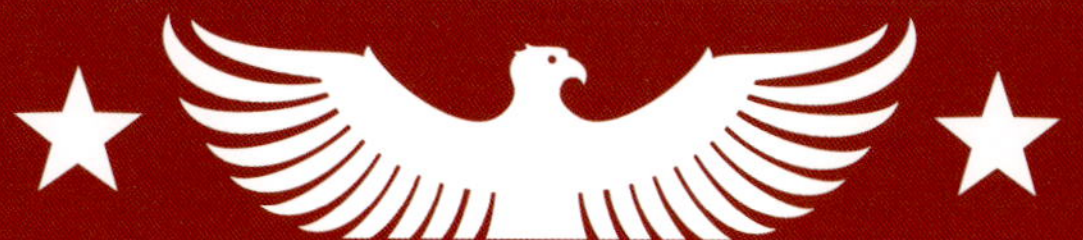

POWER • AUTHORITY • GOVERNANCE

Centers for Disease Control and Prevention

CONTENTS

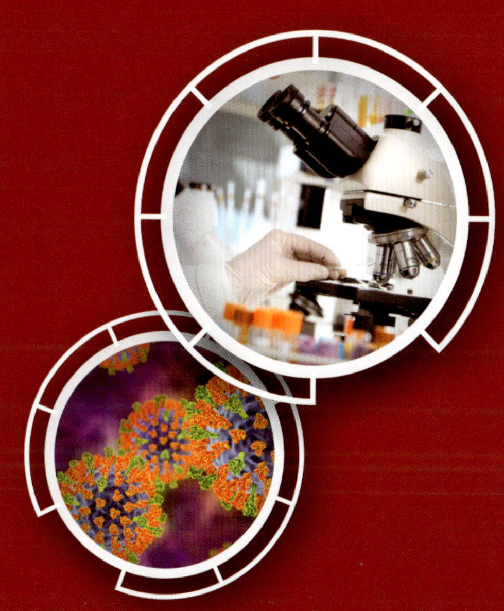

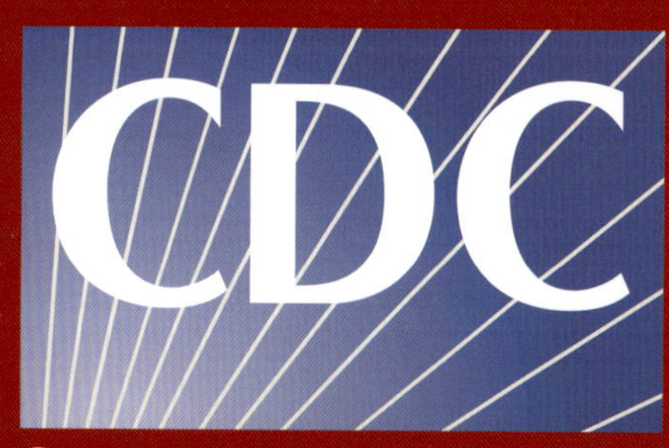

CENTERS FOR DISEASE CONTROL AND PREVENTION

Introduction

The Centers for Disease Control and Prevention (CDC) is the leading public health agency in the United States. This federal agency is committed to protecting the health, safety, and security of all Americans. The CDC is a key component of the Department of Health and Human Services. It focuses specifically on preventing and controlling disease.

The CDC was formed more than 70 years ago to help stop the spread of a disease called **malaria**. Over time, the agency's work expanded to combat other diseases as well. Today, the CDC works tirelessly to protect the nation from any disease, no matter what type of illness it is or where it comes from.

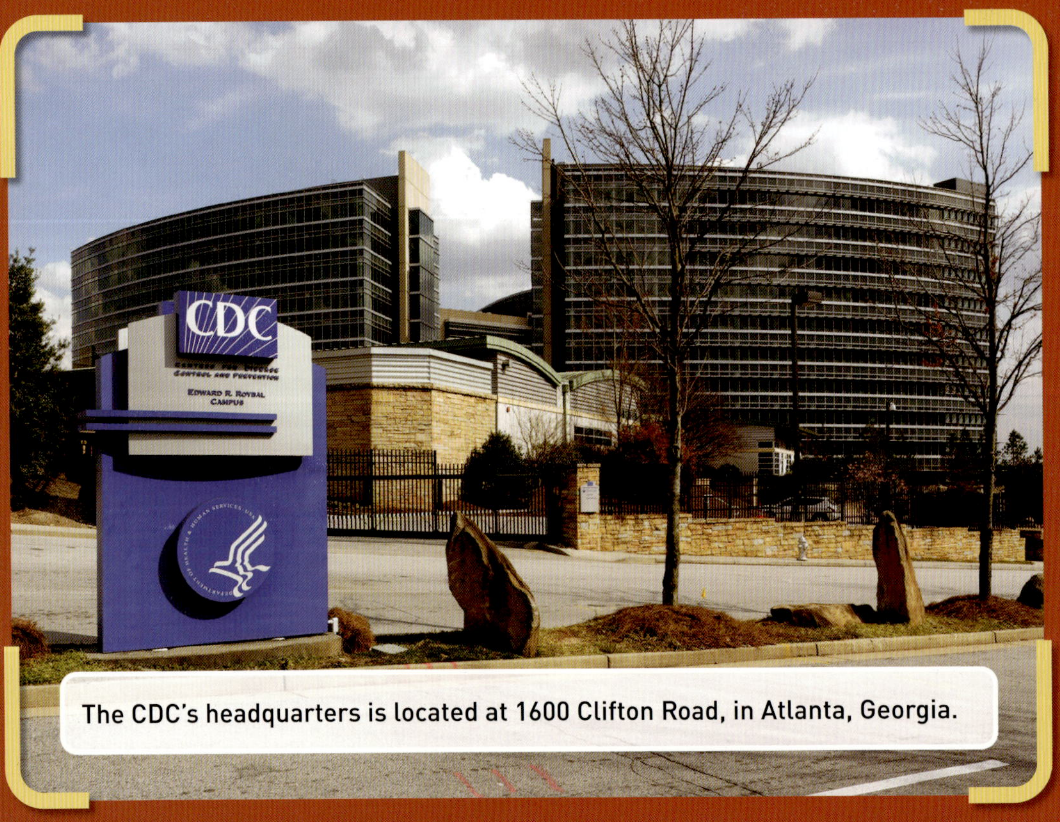

The CDC's headquarters is located at 1600 Clifton Road, in Atlanta, Georgia.

Science and data are crucial to the CDC's work. The CDC shares important health information with communities and citizens around the country. It also works to detect, track, and respond to health threats. This work increases the health security of the nation and helps people live healthier, safer lives.

The U.S. government is based on the idea of "popular sovereignty." This means that the government's power and authority come from the people of the United States. The federal government and its agencies, including the CDC, must carry out their work in accordance with the U.S. **Constitution**. As public health is not specifically mentioned in the U.S. Constitution, many public health activities are the responsibility of the states themselves.

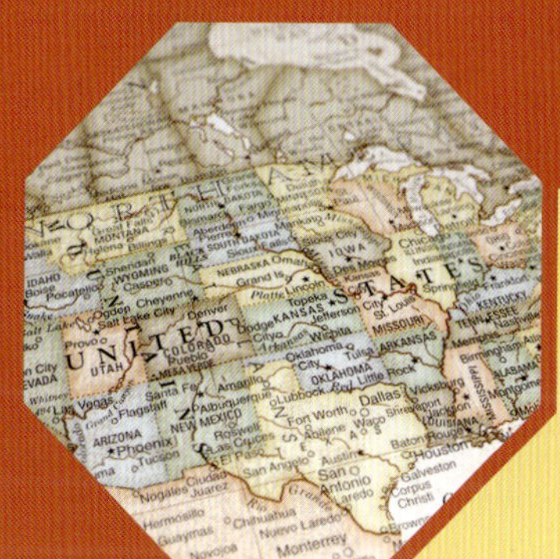

The **CDC has workers** in all **50 states**.

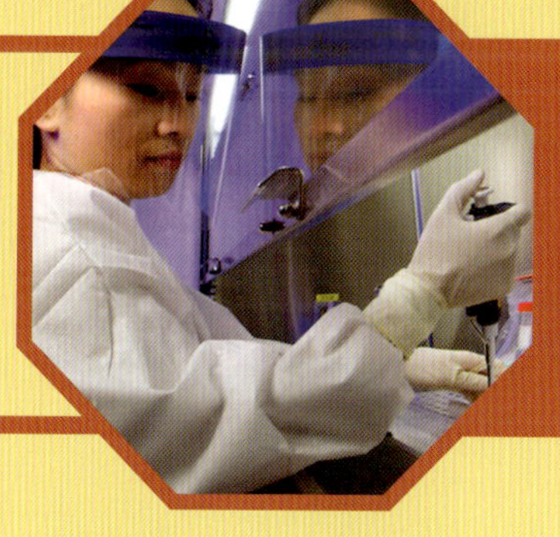

More than **200** specialized **CDC laboratories** are **spread across** the **United States**.

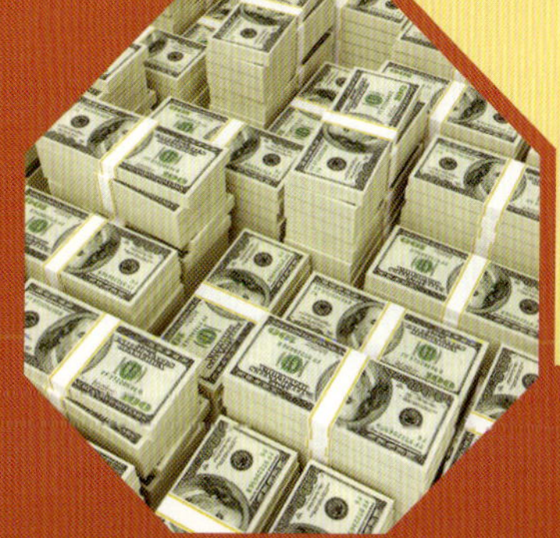

When the CDC launched in **1946**, its **budget** was only **$10 million**. In **2020**, it was more than **$6.5 billion**.

Origins of the CDC

The origins of the CDC date back to July 1, 1946, when an organization known as the Communicable Disease Center first opened its doors. This CDC was initially solely focused on stopping the spread of malaria across the United States. While many government agencies were based in Washington, DC, the CDC was located in Atlanta, Georgia, because most malaria transmission at the time was occurring in the South. The organization focused on controlling the mosquitoes that spread the disease.

By 1951, malaria was considered eliminated from the United States. However, the CDC's focus had already expanded to include all communicable diseases. These are diseases that can spread from one person or animal to another. Disease **surveillance** became an important part of the CDC's work. The center also began to help state health departments when needed.

As the CDC continued to grow, so did its responsibilities. In 1970, its name was changed to the Center for Disease Control. This change in name reflected the expansion of its work into other health areas, such as environmental health and **chronic** diseases. In 1980, the center was reorganized and renamed again, becoming the Centers for Disease Control. Health education and the promotion of good health became more important to the agency's mission around this time. In the following decade, the CDC increased its focus on preventing health problems related to disease, disability, and injury. In 1992, it was renamed the Centers for Disease Control and Prevention, which it is still known as today.

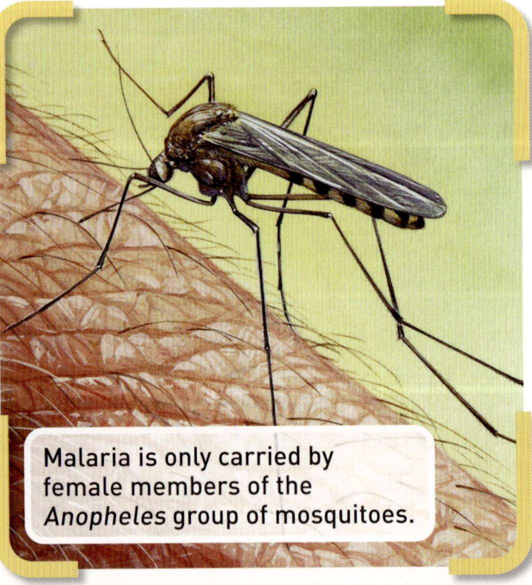

Malaria is only carried by female members of the *Anopheles* group of mosquitoes.

Branches of Government

The U.S. Constitution divides the government intro three branches. These are known as the **executive**, **legislative**, and **judicial** branches. The CDC is an agency within the executive branch of the U.S. government. This branch enforces and carries out laws. Federal agencies, committees, and departments do much of the work in the executive branch. There are many executive departments, including the U.S. Department of Health and Human Services (HHS). The CDC is one of many agencies within this department.

The division of government ensures that no person or group has too much power. Each branch has certain powers and the ability to respond to actions of the other branches. This is called a system of checks and balances. Congress, the legislative branch, is responsible for creating laws. It is also in charge of the annual federal budget. Every year, federal agencies send budget requests to the White House. These requests are used to develop the president's budget proposal, which is submitted to Congress for review. Through this process, Congress controls funding to the CDC and other agencies. The judicial branch ensures that the other branches follow the law.

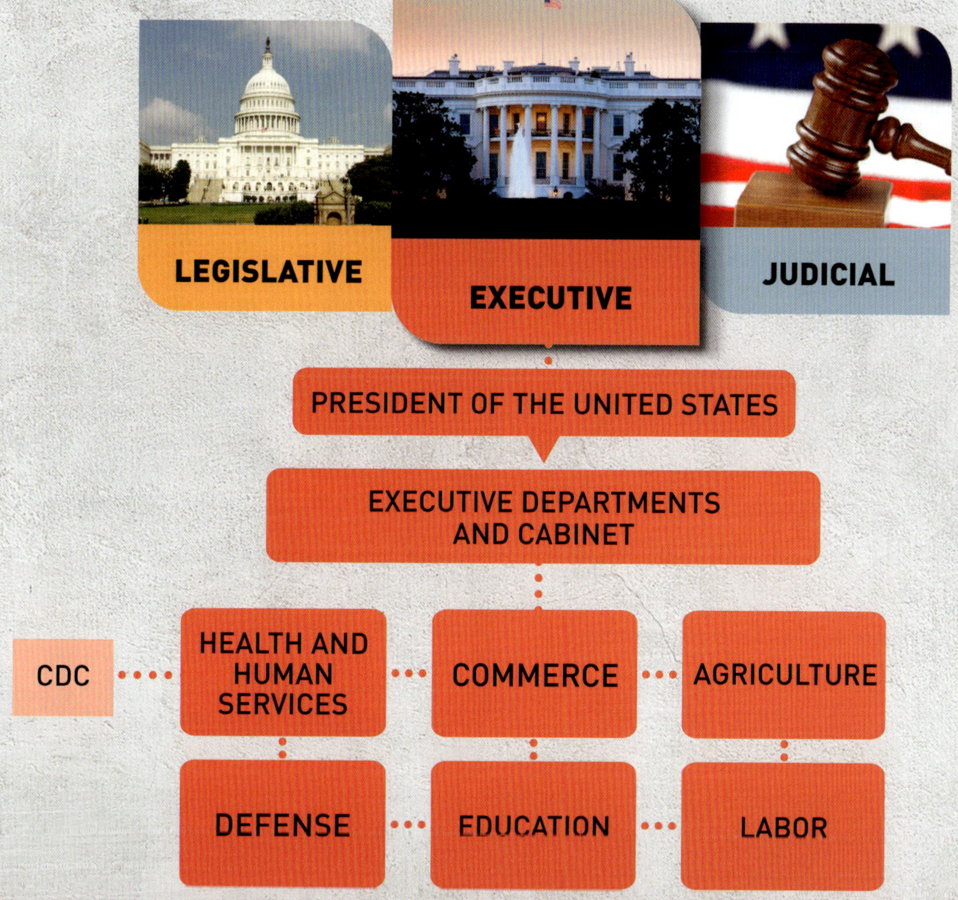

Purpose of the CDC

The CDC is a service organization. It is based in science and driven by data. The CDC's work is centered around three key areas. These are securing global health and America's preparedness, ending epidemics, and eliminating disease.

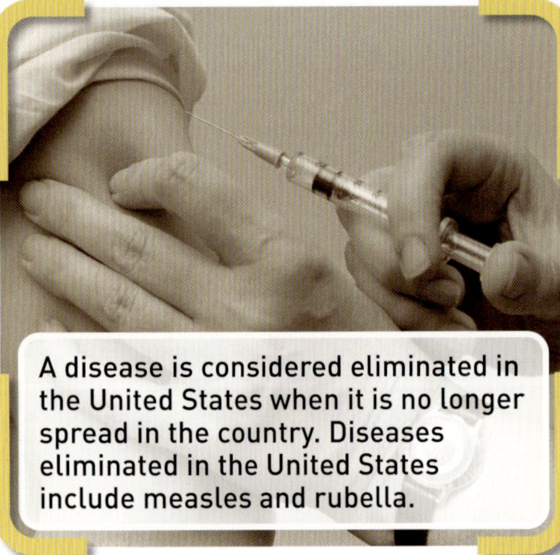

A disease is considered eliminated in the United States when it is no longer spread in the country. Diseases eliminated in the United States include measles and rubella.

The CDC secures global health and America's preparedness in many different ways. This work includes helping to stop the spread of diseases and **contagions** both at home and abroad, supporting U.S. public health **infrastructure**, and preventing **bioterrorism** threats.

Ending epidemics is an ambitious goal for the CDC. A disease is considered an epidemic when it affects a large number of people within a certain community or region at the same time. When epidemics occur, the CDC works to detect them and address the problem as quickly as possible. This includes working to prevent and control **seasonal influenza,** eliminating or reducing diseases such as HIV and type 2 diabetes, and fighting the spread of more recent illnesses, such as COVID-19.

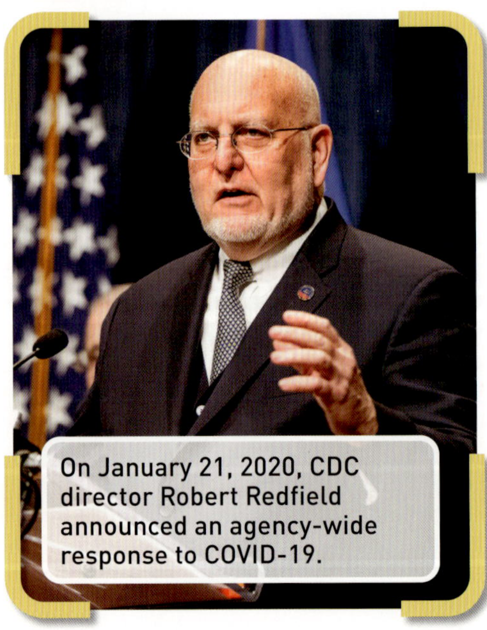

On January 21, 2020, CDC director Robert Redfield announced an agency-wide response to COVID-19.

The third area of focus for the CDC is eliminating disease. The CDC provides leadership in this area both across the country and internationally. This area of work includes **vaccination** programs and policies, initiatives to reduce chronic disease and death related to causes such as tobacco use, and efforts to reduce health problems in pregnant women.

Global Health Security Agenda

As the world becomes more connected, with many people and goods traveling internationally, infectious diseases can quickly spread from one country to another. By helping to fight global health threats, the United States also protects itself. Having strong public health systems in place to prevent, detect, and respond to diseases around the world is an important way to ensure global health security.

The Global Health Security Agenda (GHSA) is an international effort by more than 70 countries to reduce the risk of infectious disease outbreaks and strengthen public health systems around the world. The CDC is one major U.S. agency that works closely with the GHSA and government partners in other countries toward the common goal of global health security.

CDC Through the Years

For more than 70 years, the CDC has been fighting diseases to help keep Americans healthy and safe. Although the CDC has changed through the years, it remains an important part of the U.S. government to this day.

July 1, 1946

The Communicable Disease Center is established. The new organization continues the work of the Malaria Control in War Areas program, which was launched several years earlier to help prevent the spread of malaria during World War II.

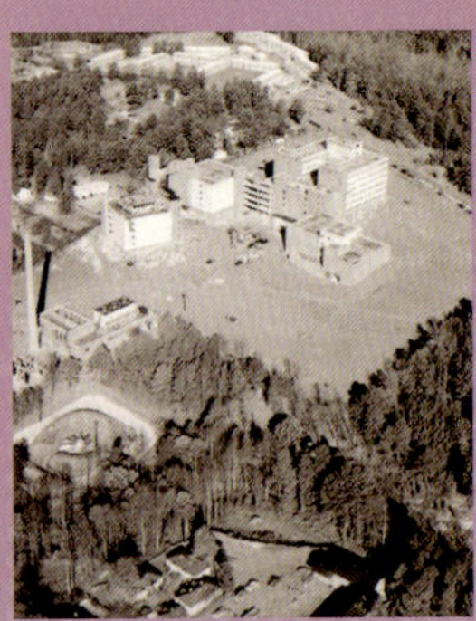

1947

The CDC pays a token $10 to Atlanta's Emory University for 15 acres (6 hectares) of land that will become the CDC headquarters.

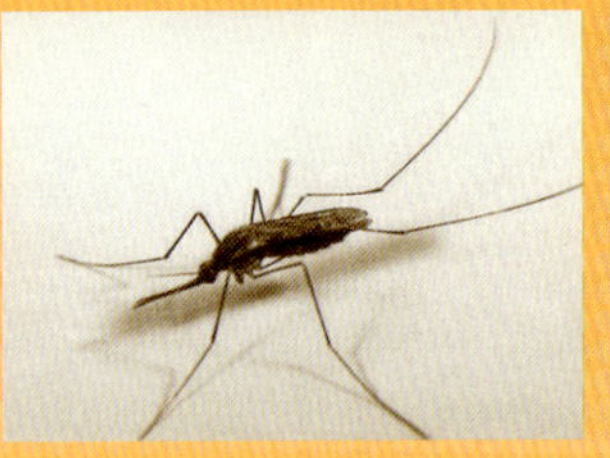

1951

Malaria is eliminated from the United States.

1960

The first National Health Examination Survey begins. Over two years, it collects data on certain chronic diseases and assesses the health of Americans across the nation.

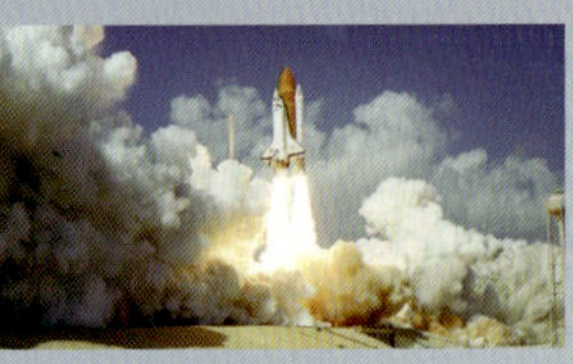

1964

The CDC works with the National Aeronautics and Space Administration (NASA) to help ensure contaminants from space do not spread on Earth after rocket and shuttle launches.

1969

The CDC opens its first permanent biological containment lab. This is meant to protect scientists that are working with dangerous **pathogens**.

1970

The U.S. Nutrition Program becomes part of the CDC. Its goal is to reduce **malnutrition** both around the world and in the United States.

1986

The Office of Smoking and Health becomes part of the CDC. It focuses on preventing health problems related to tobacco use.

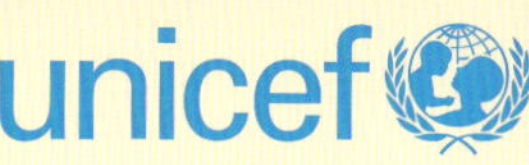

1988

The Global Polio Eradication Initiative is launched. The program is a public-private partnership between national governments and organizations including **UNICEF**, the World Health Organization (WHO), and the CDC.

1988

The CDC's Center for Chronic Disease Prevention and Health Promotion is established to help prevent diseases such as cancer and diabetes.

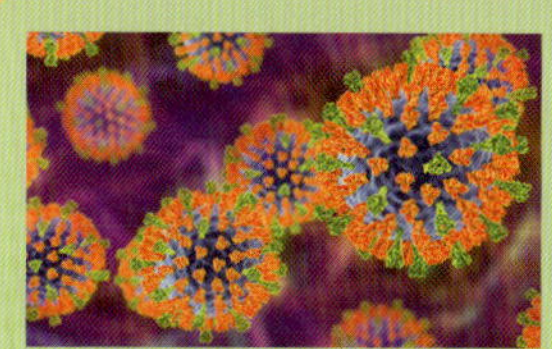

1994

The Vaccines for Children Program is put into action. This program provides vaccines at no cost to eligible children in order to help protect against diseases.

2000

Measles is declared eliminated from the United States.

2012

The CDC responds to an outbreak of an infection called fungal meningitis. At the time, it is the one of the largest healthcare-associated outbreaks in U.S. history.

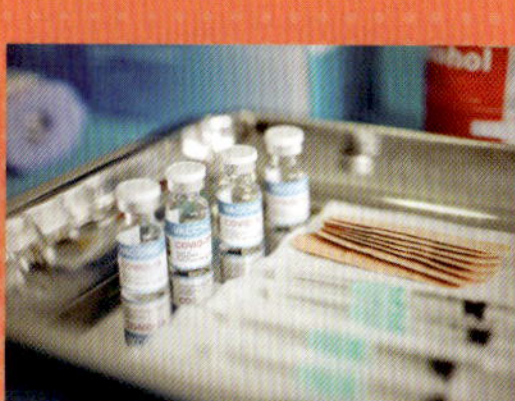

2021

More than 7,500 CDC members help the United States respond to the global COVID-19 pandemic.

CDC Issues

Threats such as disease or bioterrorism require swift and coordinated action. However, this can lead to several issues. There have been situations in which the CDC's responses to events have been considered slow, disorganized, or harmful.

Many have criticized the CDC for its involvement in the Tuskegee Study. This study began in 1932. About 600 African American men were infected with a disease. However, they did not give informed consent before this happened. This means that the researchers did not properly inform the men about the study's true purpose. As part of the study, the men were also not given proper treatment for the disease. An advisory panel concluded that the study was unethical, and it was stopped in 1972. In 1973, survivors were awarded reparations. Following the Tuskagee Study, the government changed its research practices. The National Research Act became law in 1974, paving the way for new standards and regulations to ensure more ethical research.

Years later, the CDC was criticized for its disorganized response to a bioterrorism incident that occurred in 2001. Anonymous letters containing a dangerous substance were sent in the mail. Investigators struggled to identify the material. Only a few certified labs could test samples of the substance, which made the process very slow. In total, 22 people developed an infection called anthrax as a result of the suspicious mail, and 5 of them died.

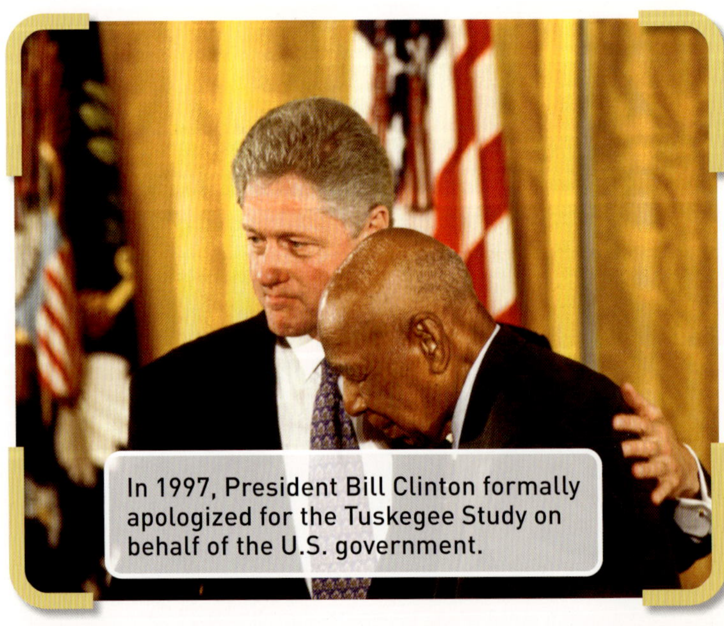

In 1997, President Bill Clinton formally apologized for the Tuskegee Study on behalf of the U.S. government.

The CDC has made changes in more recent years to address some of these concerns. It has strengthened existing programs to be better prepared for bioterrorism and other emergencies. The organization has also created rapid response teams with specialized training to respond to terrorist attacks.

Federal Rules and Regulations

The CDC has the authority to develop certain regulations or "rules" that increase public health security or help protect the United States from health or safety threats. When a Congressional bill is passed into law, the CDC may need to put it into action. The organization does this by creating regulations.

In creating regulations, agencies must be careful not to violate the Constitution or go beyond their authority. Before a new rule can take effect, it must be sent to the government accountability office and Congress for review. The rule becomes void if the Senate and House disapprove and the President agrees with them, or if both houses override a presidential **veto**. Congress can also restrict funding to agencies or create new legislation. Through these checks and balances, the CDC and other federal agencies are kept **accountable**.

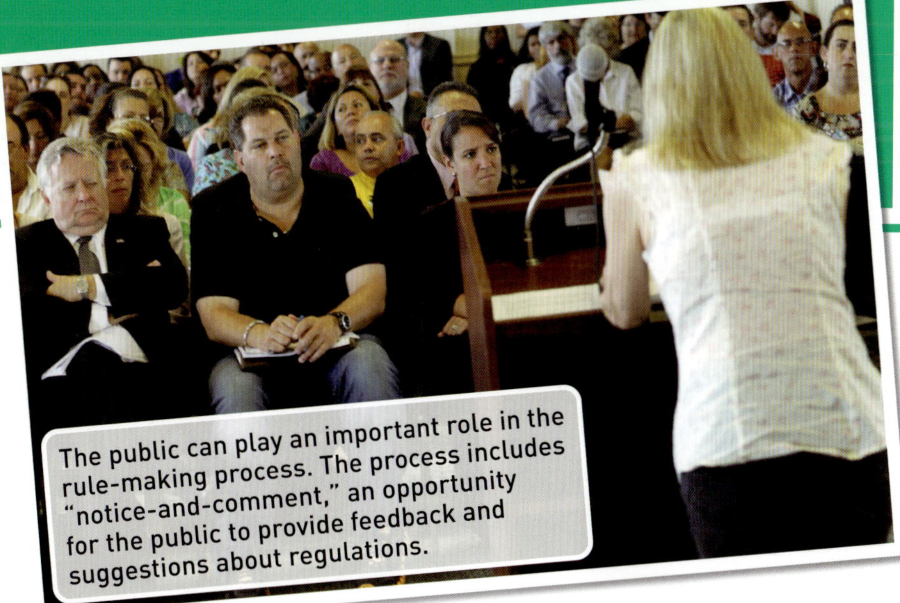

The public can play an important role in the rule-making process. The process includes "notice-and-comment," an opportunity for the public to provide feedback and suggestions about regulations.

Key Figures in the CDC

The CDC is responsible for protecting the health of millions of Americans. Key figures throughout the CDC's history have served the United States in many ways.

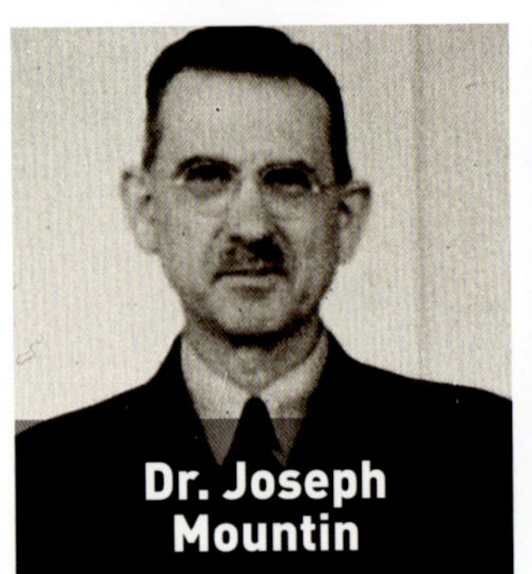

Dr. Joseph Mountin

Dr. Joseph Mountin (1891–1952) was the founder of the original CDC. He believed that the country needed an agency focused on health, disease, and environmental issues, and worked to make it a reality. His passion helped shape the CDC and the work it continues today.

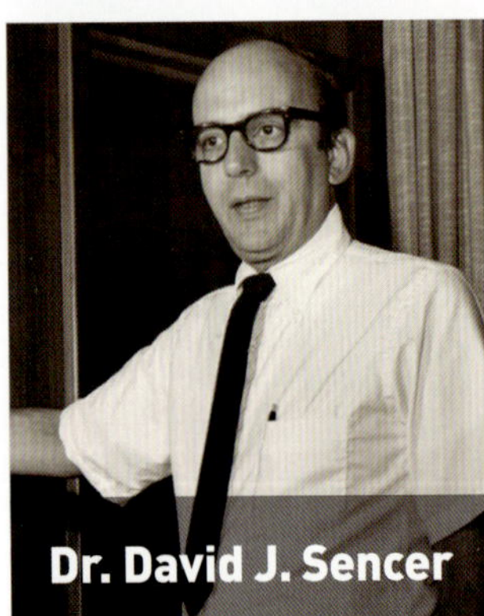

Dr. David J. Sencer

David J. Sencer (1924–2011) directed the CDC from 1966 to 1977. One of the CDC's greatest successes under his direction was the eradication of smallpox. The David J. Sencer CDC Museum in Atlanta, Georgia, was renamed in his honor in 2011.

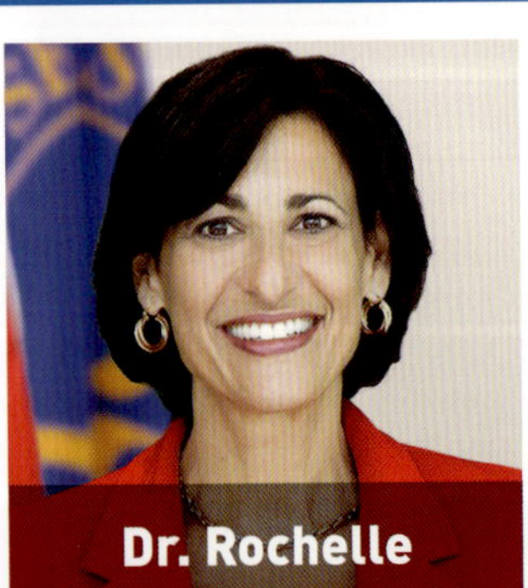

Dr. Rochelle Walensky

Dr. Rochelle Walensky (1969–) is the current director of the CDC. She was selected by President Joe Biden to lead the organization in responding to COVID-19. Prior to her role at the CDC, Dr. Walensky worked as both a physician and researcher.

Polio

HISTORICAL CASE STUDY

Poliomyelitis, also known as polio, is a disease caused by the poliovirus. In the 1950s, it was one of the most feared diseases in the United States. Polio is very contagious, and it mainly affects children. It can damage the spinal cord and brain, leading to paralysis.

The virus reached its peak in the United States in 1952, infecting about 60,000 people. After years of research, a vaccine was released in 1955. Vaccinations began immediately. However, within just a few days, a child who had received the vaccine was diagnosed with polio.

Additional cases soon emerged, raising questions about the vaccine. The CDC's Epidemic Intelligence Service (EIS) was called in to investigate. The EIS was a group of epidemiologists trained to respond to emergencies. EIS created a national surveillance system and traced 260 cases to unsafe vaccines. The CDC was able to confirm that all cases were linked to vaccines from one manufacturer. The other manufacturers were cleared to continue producing vaccines, and the vaccination program could resume. Public confidence in the program was regained. As a result, polio cases declined, and vaccine safety controls were improved.

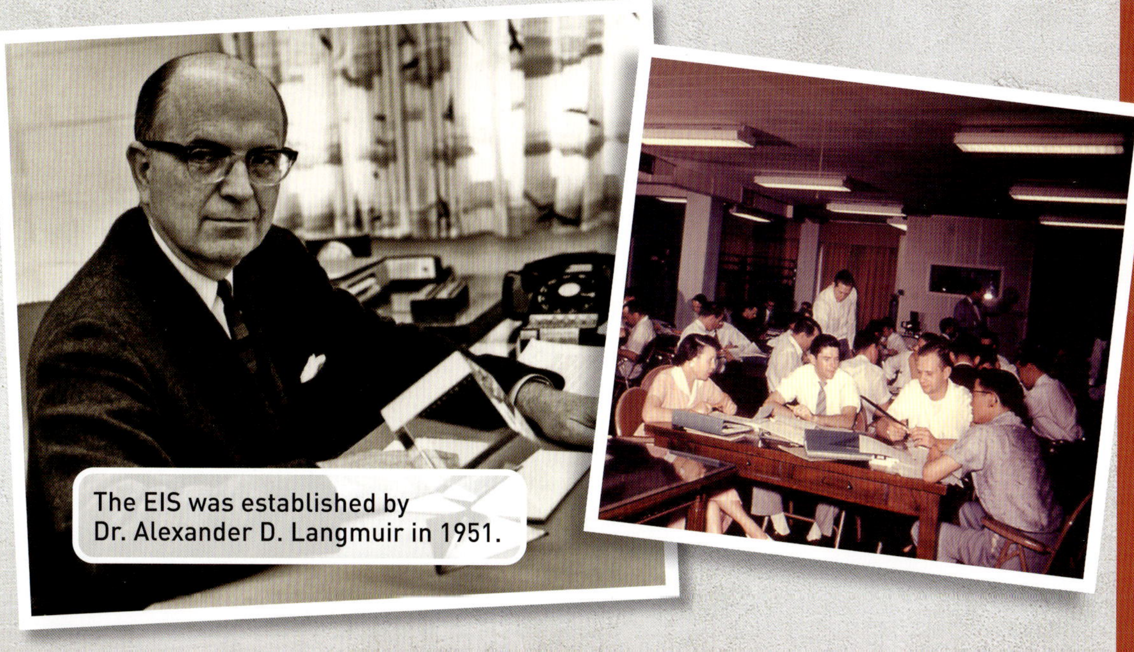

The EIS was established by Dr. Alexander D. Langmuir in 1951.

Careers in the CDC

Emergency Management Specialist

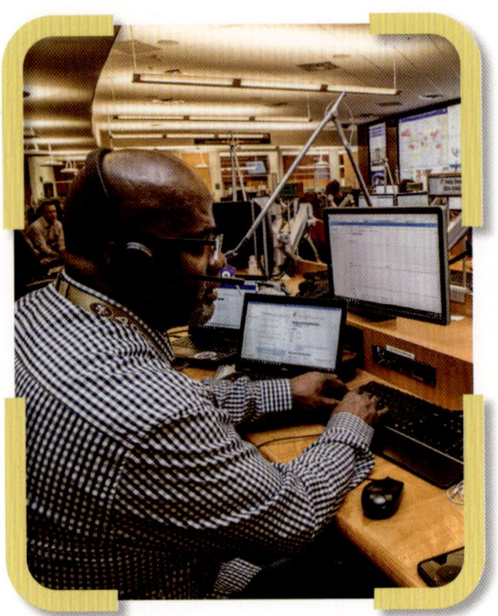

Emergency Management Specialists at the CDC may take on many different roles. One is to make sure the CDC is prepared for emergencies. Workers in this role also evaluate how the agency has performed when responding to an emergency and identify ways to improve responses for the future. Strong organization and communication skills are important to success in this type of role.

Epidemiologist

Epidemiologists look for clues, such as who is getting sick and what symptoms they have, to find the cause of a disease, determine how to control its spread, and prevent future reoccurrence. Epidemiologists must have strong skills in math and statistics. This job requires a master's degree or higher education.

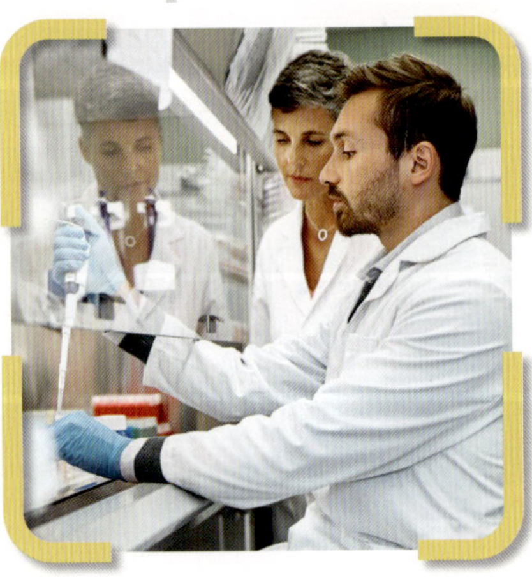

Health Scientist

The role of a health scientist is to provide scientific advice and find solutions to health problems. These scientists plan and conduct research. They may also help to develop materials to teach people about diseases and other health topics. Some colleges offer a specific health science degree program.

Medical Officer

Medical officers work in many areas, including research, scientific investigations, serving as advisors and consultants, and working with CDC partners to provide specialized services. A career in this area is best suited to someone who enjoys science and has an interest in supporting public health.

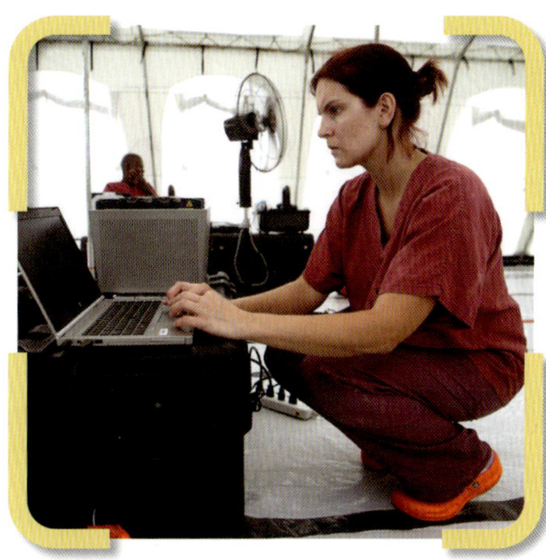

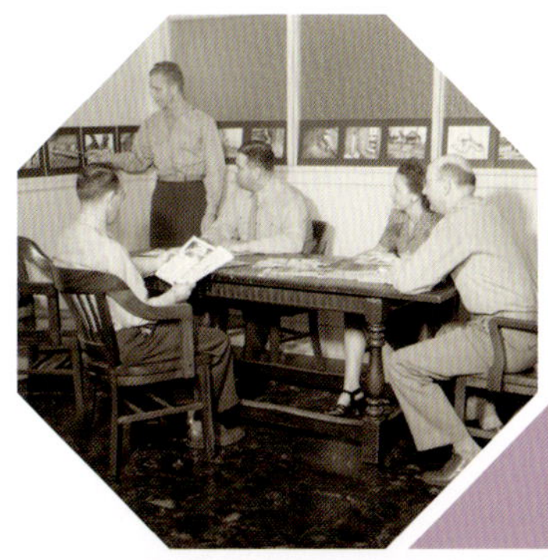

Since its beginning in **1946**, more than **50,000** people have **worked** at the CDC.

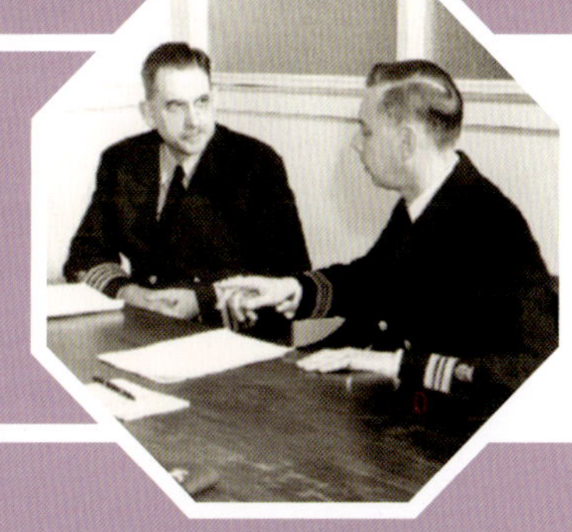

Of the original **369** CDC staff, **only 7** were **medical officers**.

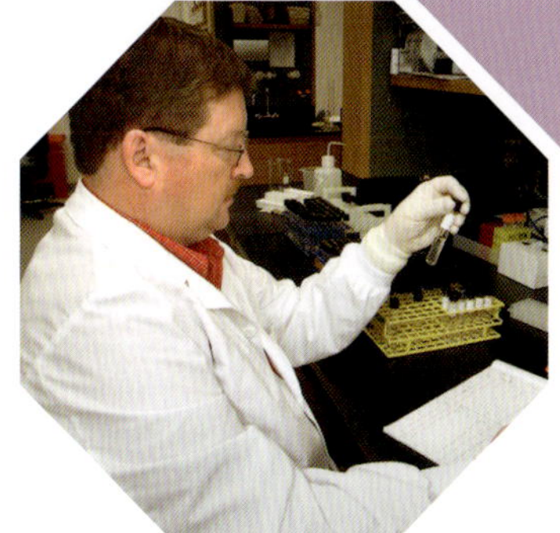

STEM stands for **Science**, **Technology**, **Engineering**, and **Math**. Nearly all careers at the CDC relate to one or more **STEM fields**.

Tools of the Trade

The CDC needs many different tools and devices to do its job. Along with examining viruses, the organization needs to be able to communicate effectively.

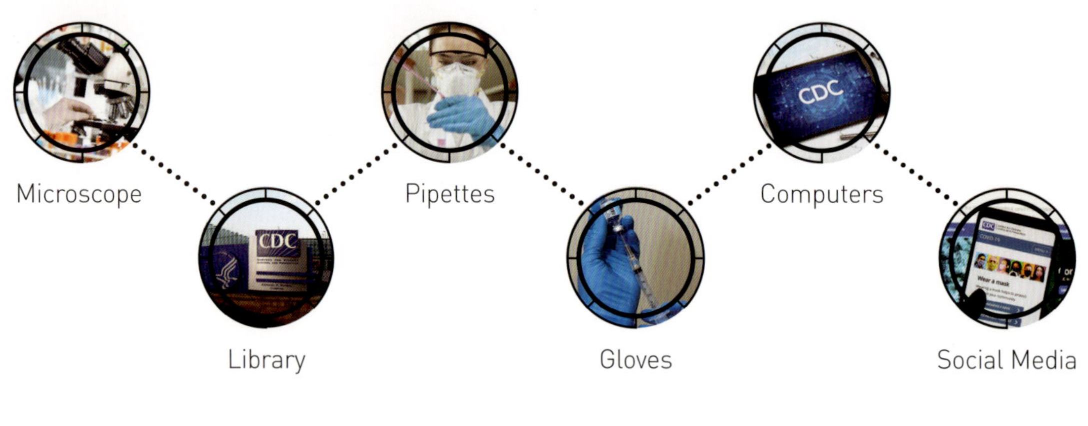

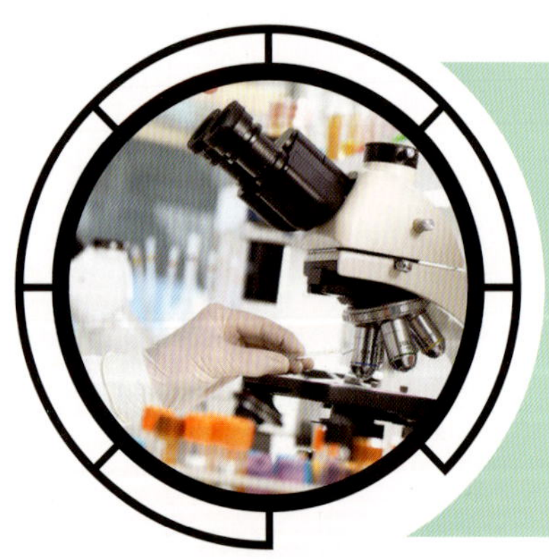

Microscope

A common piece of equipment used in laboratories is a microscope. Microscopes magnify very small objects to help scientists view them. In CDC microbiology labs, workers must know how to use a bright field, or compound, microscope. This type of microscope has two or more lenses and creates a dark image against a bright background.

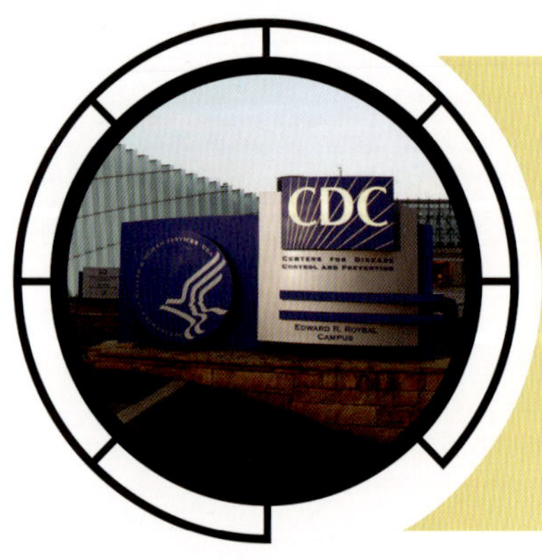

Library

The CDC has its own specialized library that supports research and learning for its employees. Named the Stephen B. Thacker CDC Library, this resource is an invaluable tool for CDC workers. Its collection covers many topics relating to public health. The library's main branch is located in the CDC's Atlanta headquarters.

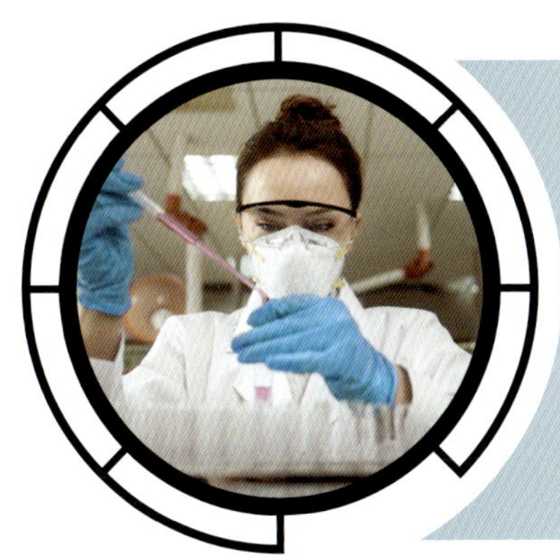

Pipettes

A pipette is a small piece of equipment used in labs to measure liquids. It can also be used to transfer liquid from one container to another. Versions have existed since the 1700s, and they remain common in laboratories today. The CDC uses pipettes to transfer and hold materials that are being tested.

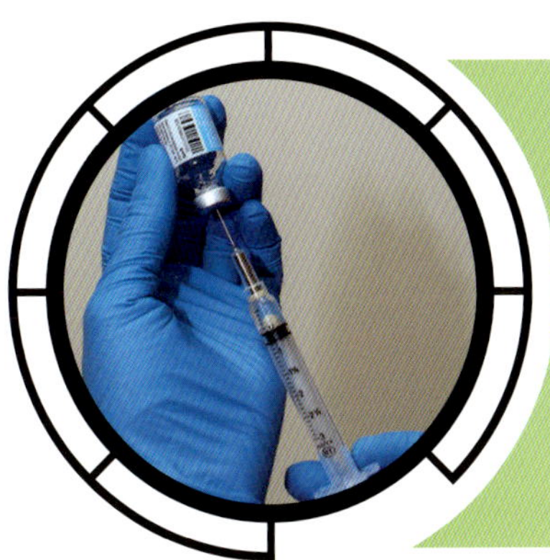

Gloves

Gloves are the most common type of Personal Protective Equipment (PPE) used by workers in a healthcare setting. Workers often use heavy latex gloves to protect their hands when they disinfect surfaces. Sterile surgical gloves are worn when medical workers treat patients.

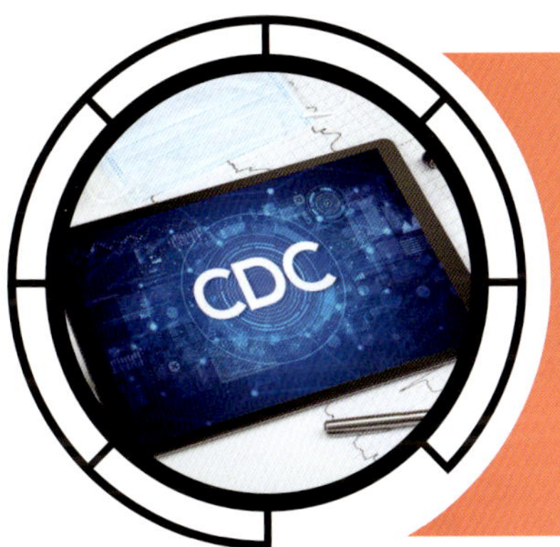

Computers

Computers are needed for much of the work done by the CDC. Computers help workers in many different roles to collect, store, and interpret data. When working in the field, CDC workers may also use personal devices such as smartphones. These devices help increase the speed and accuracy of health data collection.

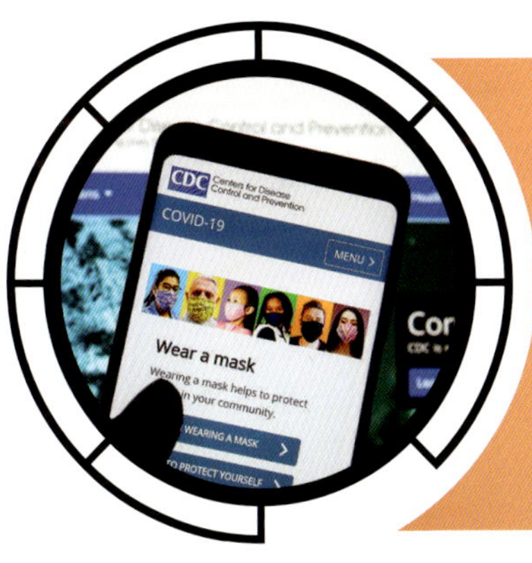

Social Media

Social media is an important tool used by the CDC to communicate health information. It includes websites and apps that allow users to quickly share stories, photos, or other information. The CDC has a presence on many different social media platforms, including YouTube, TikTok, Facebook, Instagram, and Pinterest.

CDC in the United States

The CDC has more than two dozen units in total. These are called the CDC's Centers, Institutes, and Offices (CIOs). Each CIO has its own area of focus or expertise.

1 Atlanta, Georgia

The CDC's headquarters opened with six buildings on September 8, 1960. It continued to grow over time. A new, expanded campus, including an updated headquarters building, opened in 2005. Originally built in an unincorporated area, the headquarters became part of the City of Atlanta in early 2018 by request of the CDC.

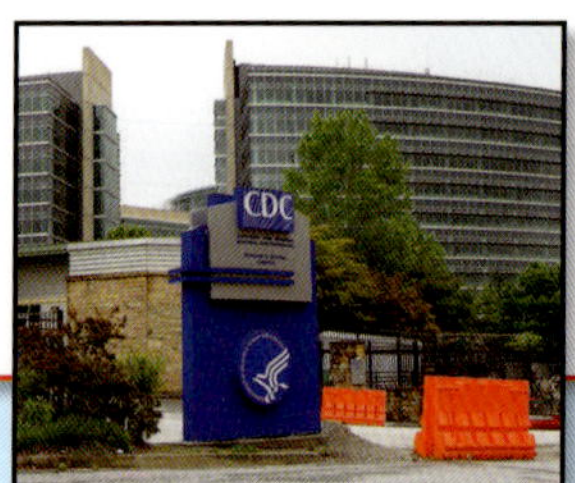

2 Fort Collins, Colorado

The Division of Vector-Borne Diseases (DVBD) works to protect people from diseases carried by vectors, such as ticks and fleas. DVBD is the CDC's only major infectious disease laboratory located outside of Atlanta. Some of the pathogens in its collection are more than 100 years old.

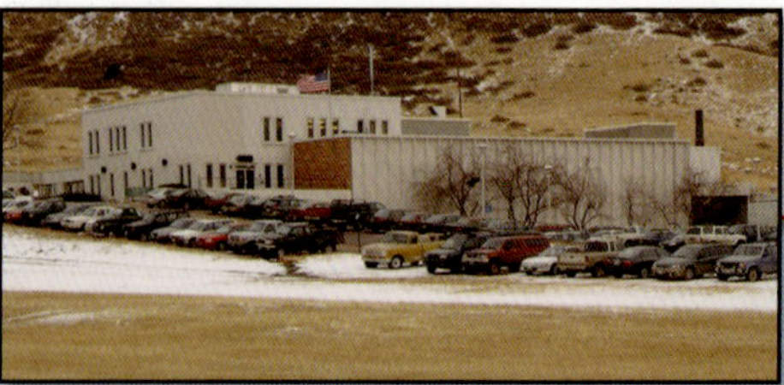

Washington
Montana
Oregon
Idaho
Wyoming
Nevada
Utah
Colorado
California
Arizona
New Mexico

LEGEND

- Land (USA)
- Land (Other)
- Water

SCALE

700 KILOMETERS
350 MILES

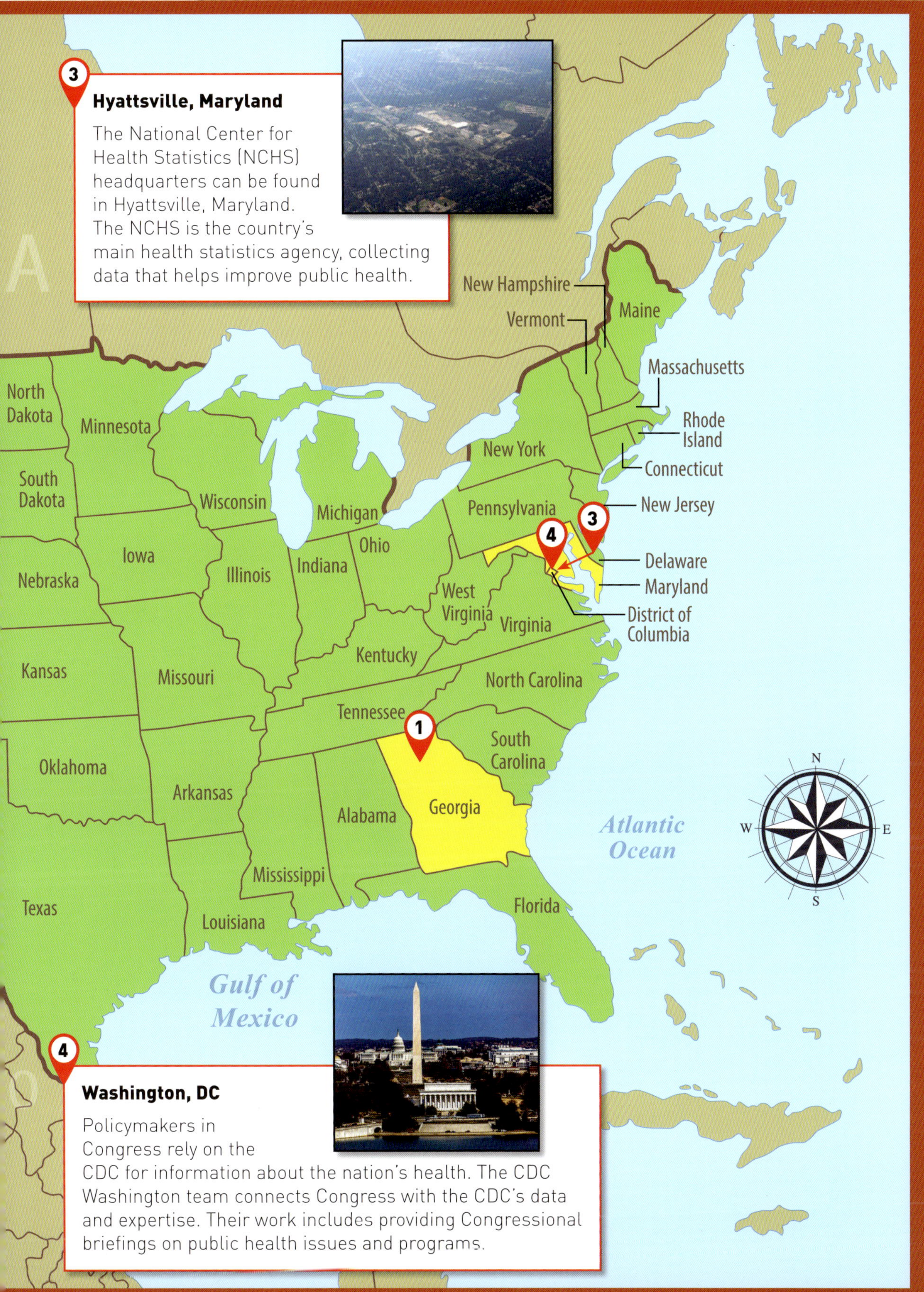

3 Hyattsville, Maryland

The National Center for Health Statistics (NCHS) headquarters can be found in Hyattsville, Maryland. The NCHS is the country's main health statistics agency, collecting data that helps improve public health.

4 Washington, DC

Policymakers in Congress rely on the CDC for information about the nation's health. The CDC Washington team connects Congress with the CDC's data and expertise. Their work includes providing Congressional briefings on public health issues and programs.

CDC in the World

For more than 60 years, the CDC has been working all across the globe to improve the health and safety of people. By sharing its expertise and knowledge, it aims to tackle global health challenges. These efforts are coordinated by the CDC's Center for Global Health and address such challenges as malaria and the health of refugees. The CDC's global programs are run by experts in areas including disease surveillance, epidemiology, and laboratory systems. This important work improves public health services for people around the world, with programs addressing more than 400 diseases, conditions, and health threats worldwide.

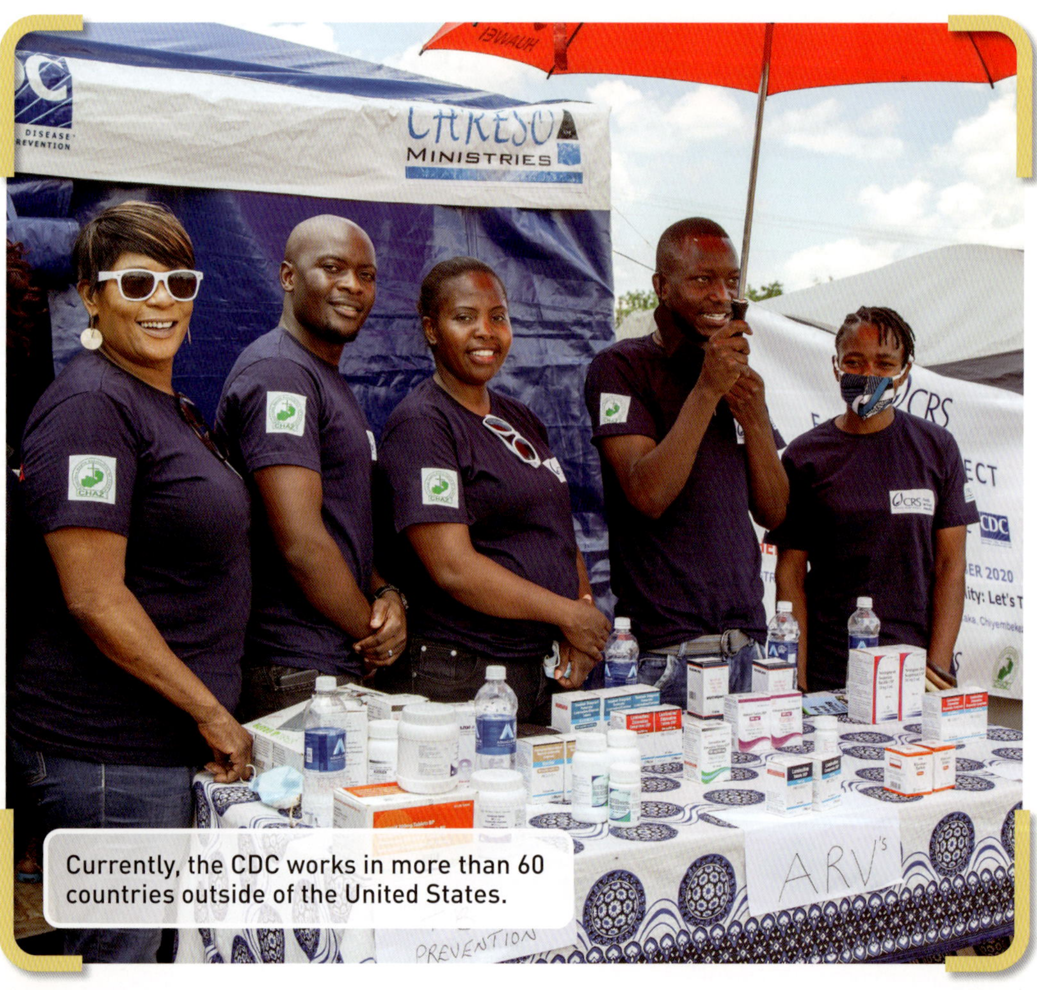

Currently, the CDC works in more than 60 countries outside of the United States.

The CDC works with many partners to tackle these challenges. These include other agencies in the U.S. government, academic institutions, foreign governments, and various non-government organizations (NGOs).

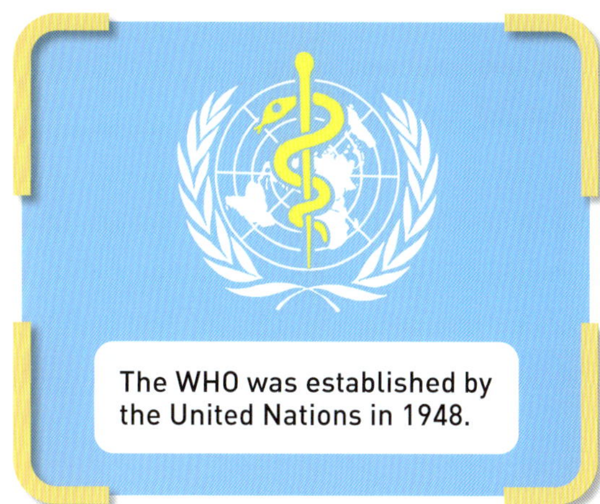

The WHO was established by the United Nations in 1948.

One of the CDC's most important partners is the WHO. The WHO is the authority on international health within the United Nations. It works with 194 member states.

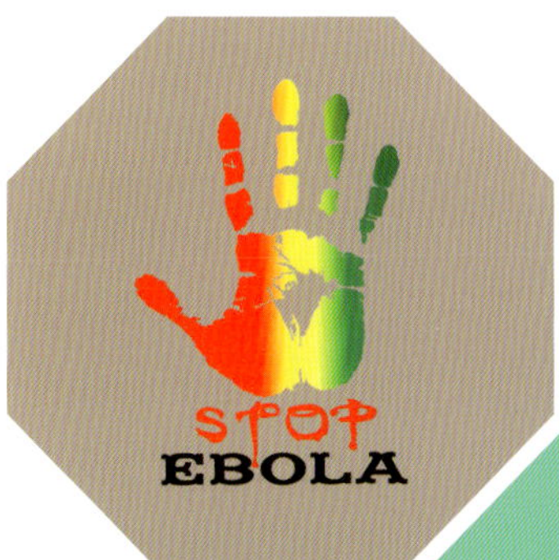

The CDC was a first responder to the **2014 Ebola outbreak** in West Africa. At the time, the outbreak was the largest of its kind in history.

Today, the WHO's goal is to provide universal health coverage for **one billion people**, protect **one billion** more from health emergencies, and provide overall better health for another **billion**.

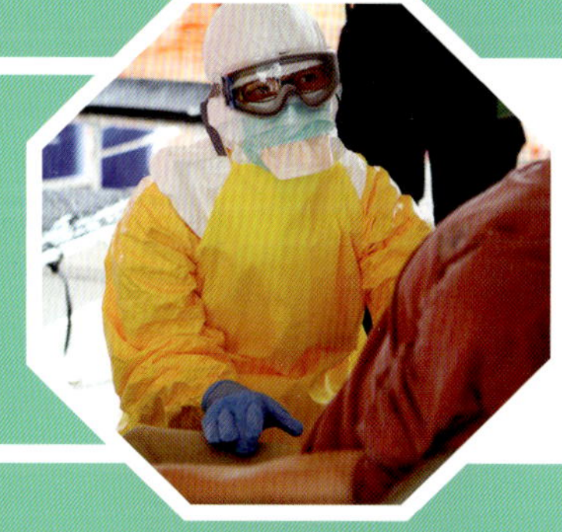

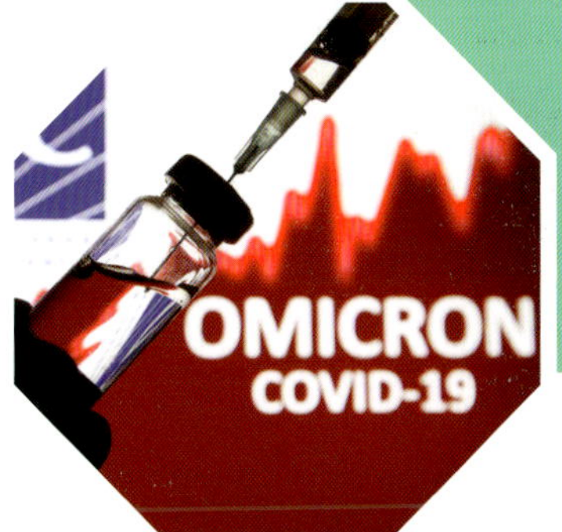

The CDC's Global Health Strategy is based on **five key pillars**. These are scientific expertise, sustainability, innovation, diverse partnerships, and equity.

CDC Today

In recent years, the CDC has been facing an enormous and challenging health crisis. The COVID-19 pandemic began in December 2019. The disease spread far and quickly, infecting people across the globe. More than 500,000 people died in the first six months. Scientists soon discovered that COVID-19 is caused by a virus now known as SARS-CoV-2.

Some have criticized the CDC's response to the pandemic for being slow and disorganized. The CDC's guidance around testing, for example, changed several times, causing doubt and confusion. Some CDC employees have suggested that the organization should be more involved in the federal strategy to prevent this confusion.

Since its initial COVID-19 response launch, the CDC has continued to learn more about the disease, including how it spreads and its impact on people and communities. The agency's response has included work in a range of areas, such as preparing healthcare providers and health systems to deal with COVID-19, providing advice to schools and businesses, protecting the health of travelers and communities, and sharing the knowledge it has gained throughout the pandemic.

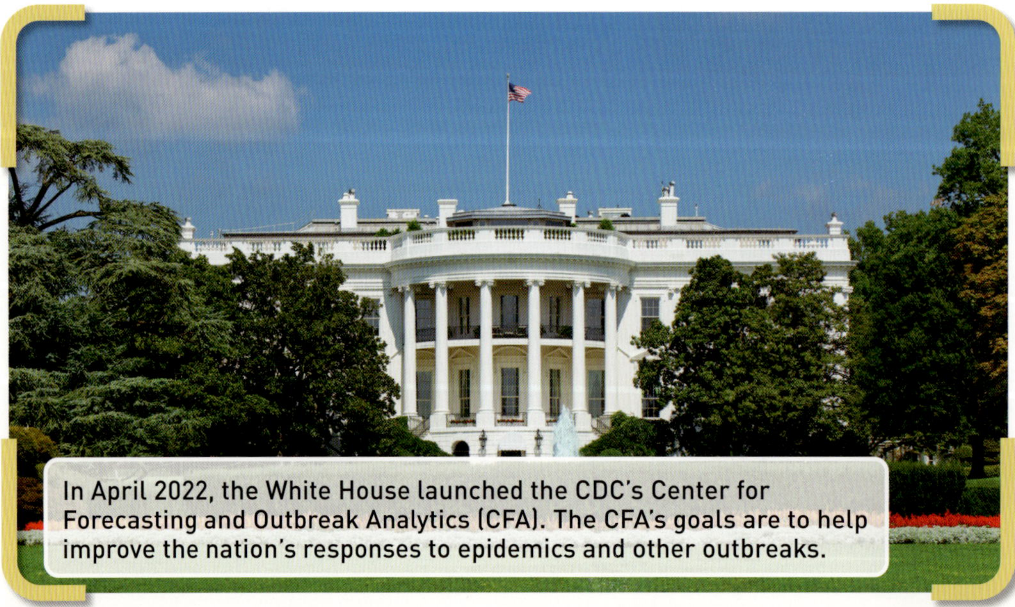

In April 2022, the White House launched the CDC's Center for Forecasting and Outbreak Analytics (CFA). The CFA's goals are to help improve the nation's responses to epidemics and other outbreaks.

Hurricane Katrina

MODERN CASE STUDY

In August 2005, Hurricane Katrina struck the United States. It killed more than 1,800 people, making it one of the largest natural disasters in the country's history.

The storm caused chaos and flooding across New Orleans. An evacuation of the city was ordered, but thousands of residents could not or would not leave their homes. Access to food and clean water became limited, while daily temperatures reached 90° Fahrenheit (32° Celsius). Floodwater became full of bacteria, causing a public health emergency.

Under the CDC's direction, a network of national centers coordinated a response. These centers trained volunteers, coordinated operation plans, sent workers and supplies to evacuation sites, and provided advice to local, state, and federal agencies. Approximately 700 CDC experts worked alongside local health workers to prevent injury, illness, and death.

Responding to a disaster of this scale offered many lessons and insights for the CDC. The agency has used these lessons to improve the way it anticipates large-scale events of this nature and become better prepared to respond to future public health emergencies.

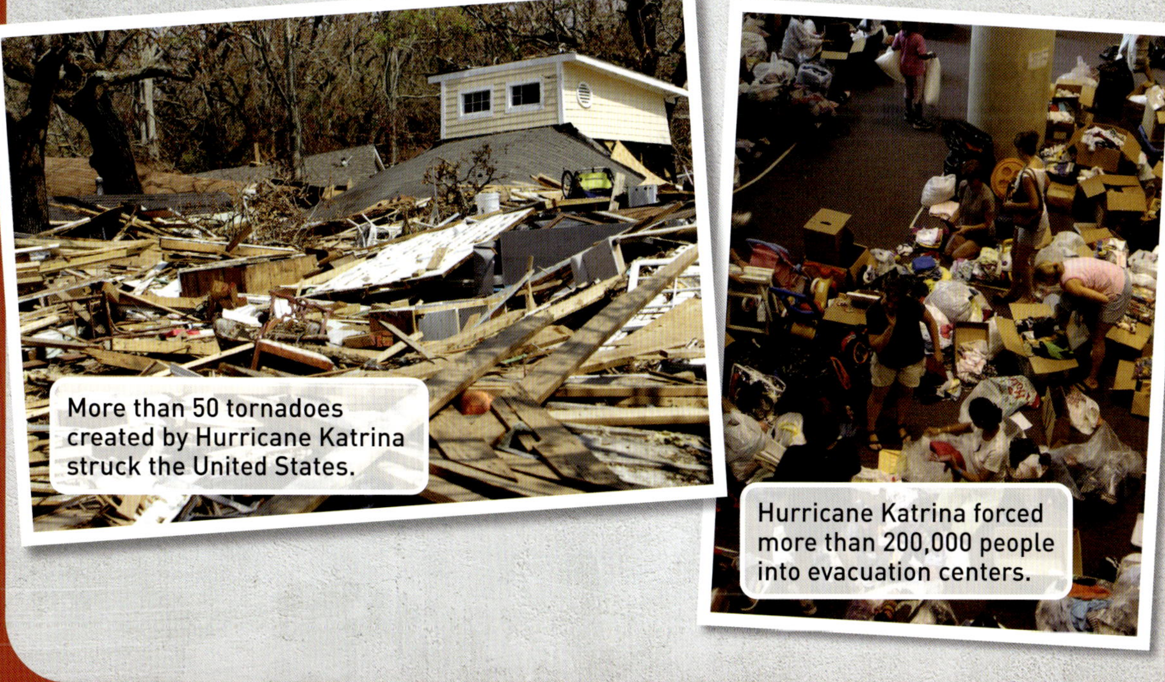

More than 50 tornadoes created by Hurricane Katrina struck the United States.

Hurricane Katrina forced more than 200,000 people into evacuation centers.

CDC Looking to the Future

Advances in technology have improved our lives in many ways, allowing people, ideas, and goods to travel around the world. As this interconnected world also creates greater opportunities for diseases to spread, the CDC must be vigilant in safeguarding the health of Americans. The COVID-19 pandemic is a devastating example of how quickly a disease can spread from one country to another. It highlights the importance of agencies like the CDC in disease surveillance, prevention, and response.

Currently, the CDC continues to face many large health challenges, such as cancer, heart disease, and other illnesses that impact millions of Americans. While some diseases have been eradicated in the United States, many continue to impact other nations around the world. Continued work by the CDC in foreign countries will remain crucial to its goal of global health security.

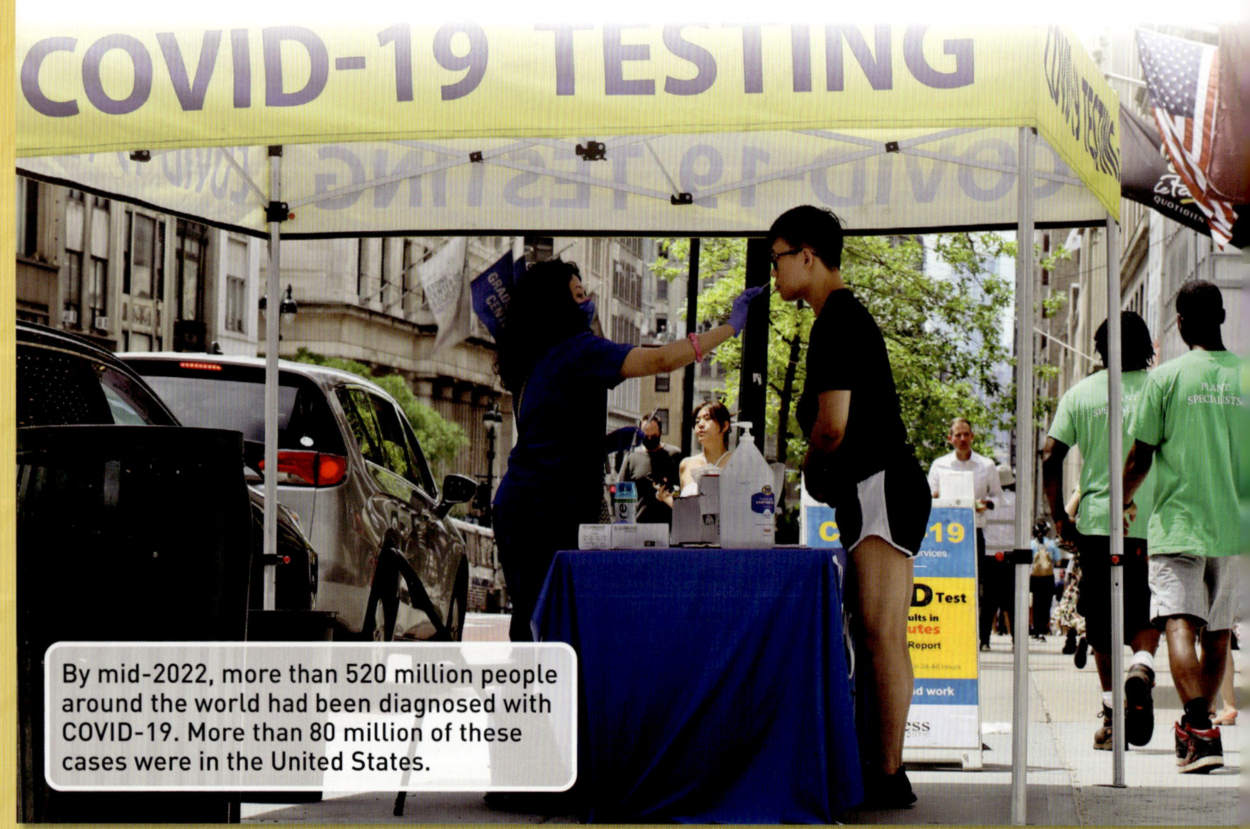

By mid-2022, more than 520 million people around the world had been diagnosed with COVID-19. More than 80 million of these cases were in the United States.

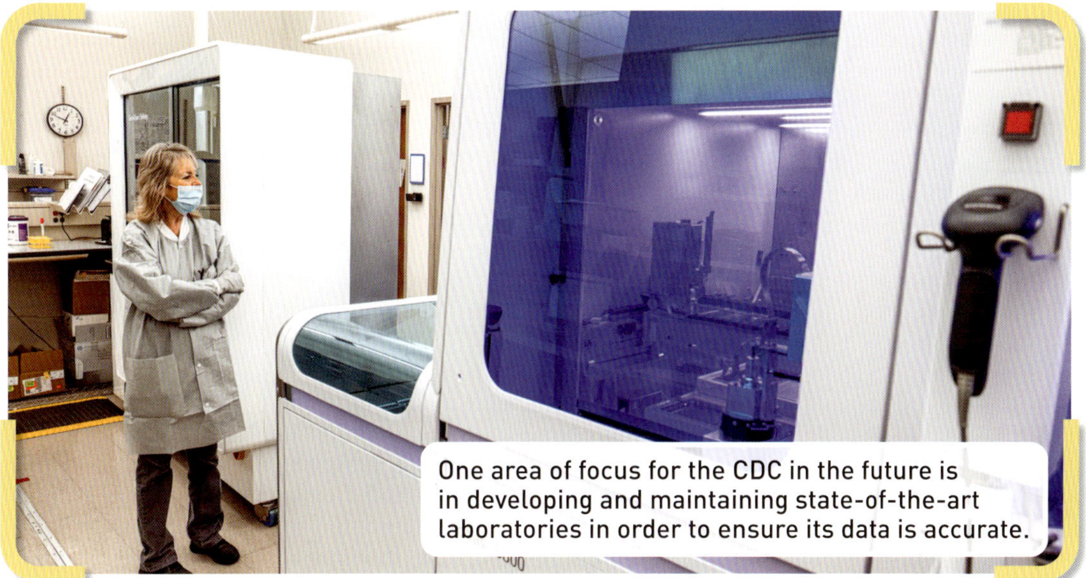

One area of focus for the CDC in the future is in developing and maintaining state-of-the-art laboratories in order to ensure its data is accurate.

Looking to the future, it is impossible to fully predict when the next natural disaster will strike or when the next disease outbreak will occur. However, the CDC will certainly play an important role in responding to these challenges and in ensuring the continued safety and health of the nation.

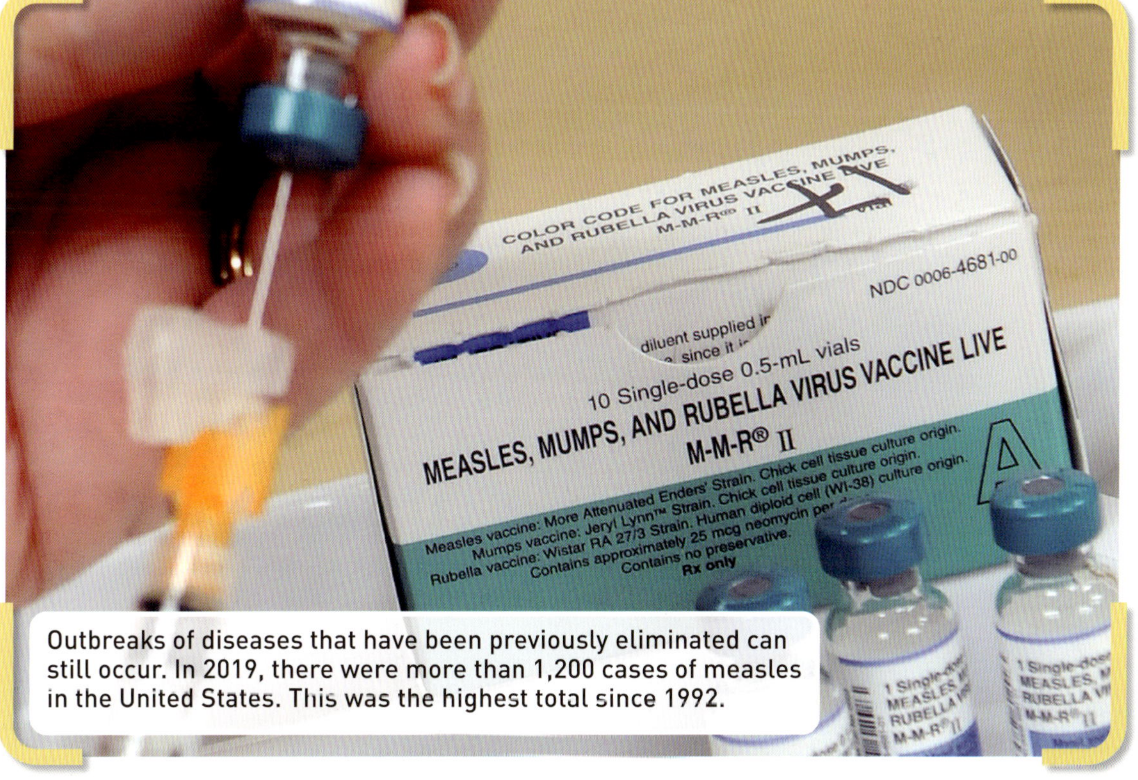

Outbreaks of diseases that have been previously eliminated can still occur. In 2019, there were more than 1,200 cases of measles in the United States. This was the highest total since 1992.

ACTIVITY ★★

Create a Policy Paper

The outbreak of a disease can be a frightening and challenging event for both government agencies and members of the public. Many people have different perspectives on what actions the government should or should not take to protect citizens during this type of event. It is important for agencies such as the CDC to balance people's safety with respecting their rights and freedoms.

Develop your own thoughts about how organizations such as the CDC should respond to an epidemic. Write a policy paper that summarizes your opinion.

Step 1:

Answer the following questions to help you develop your opinion.

1. Which is more important to you—your health and safety or your freedom? Why do you feel this way?
2. Are you willing to give up certain rights during an outbreak to help protect your family or community from the disease? Why or why not?
3. Should measures to reduce the spread of disease be voluntary or enforced by law? Why or why not?
4. Should the CDC have authority to restrict certain freedoms during an epidemic? Why or why not?
5. Should the health and well-being of individual people or society as a whole be prioritized? Why?
6. Even during a health emergency, are there certain rights the CDC should not be allowed to infringe on? Which ones and why?
7. What other factors should the CDC consider in its response to a disease outbreak?

Step 2:

Take your opinions from questions 1 to 7 and write a one-page policy paper. This should explain the policy you think would balance people's health and safety with individual rights and freedoms during an epidemic. Follow the format outlined below.

- Paragraph 1: What is the issue?
- Paragraph 2: What are the problematic points surrounding the issue?
- Paragraph 3: What is your policy on the issue, and why?

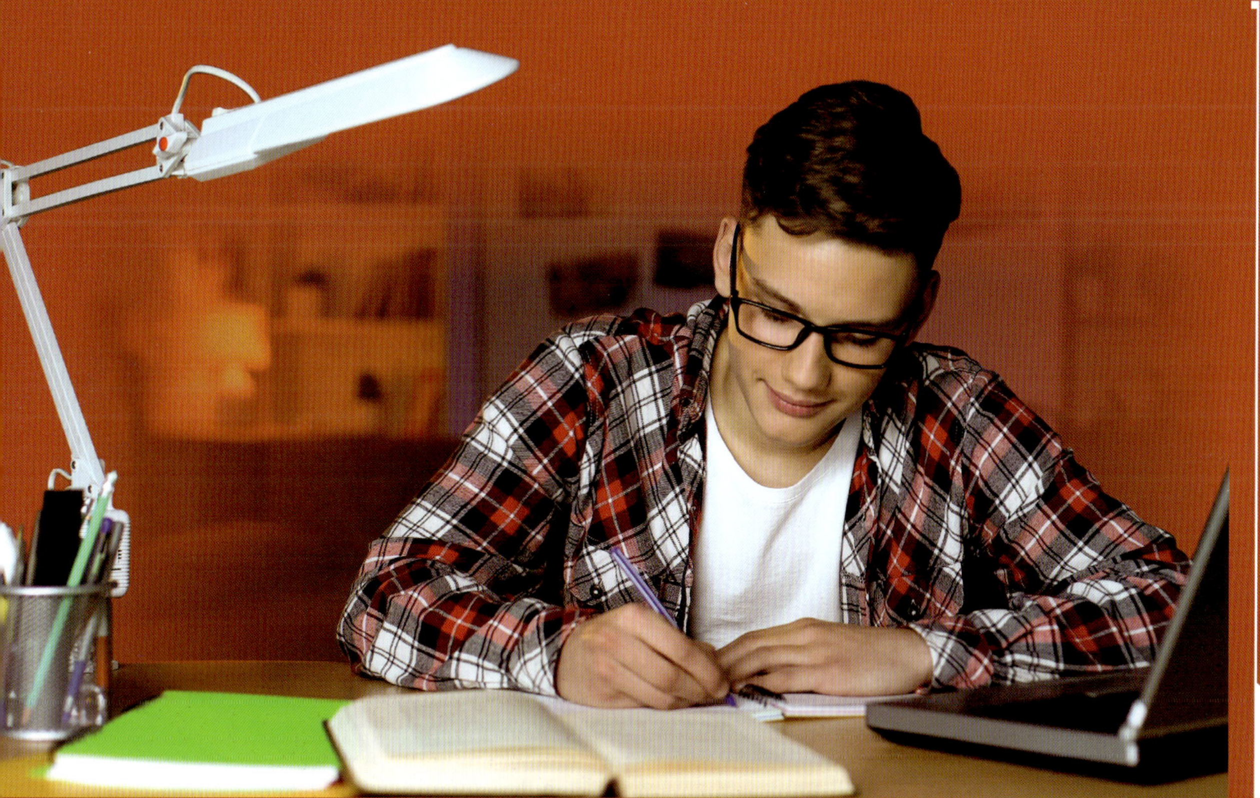

QUIZ ★★

1 In what year was the CDC established?

2 What is the CDC committed to protect?

3 Which federal department is the CDC part of?

4 Which tools are used by the CDC to magnify small objects?

5 Which CDC employees investigate the causes of diseases?

6 Who was the founder of the CDC?

7 How many different countries are part of the GHSA?

8 Where is the CDC's headquarters located?

9 In what year was measles eliminated from the United States?

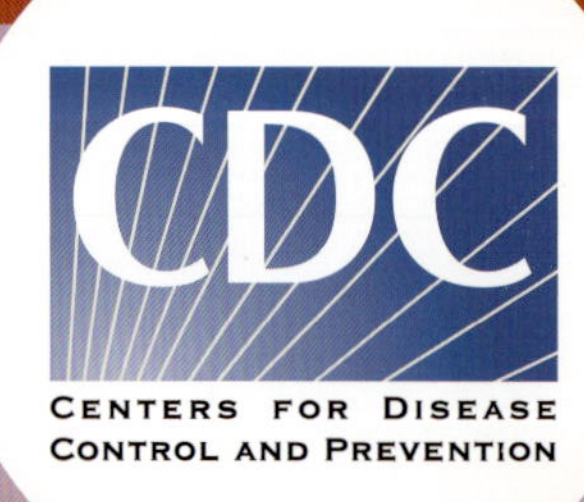

10 What major natural disaster did the CDC respond to in 2005?

ANSWERS

1. 1946 2. The health, safety, and security of Americans 3. U.S. Department of Health and Human Services 4. Microscopes 5. Epidemiologists 6. Dr. Joseph Mountin 7. More than 70 8. Atlanta, Georgia 9. 2000 10. Hurricane Katrina

KEY WORDS

accountable: when someone or something is held responsible for its actions

bioterrorism: violent action using living material, such as bacteria, to harm or kill people for political motives

chronic: something that continues or occurs again and again, for a long time

constitution: a country's basic laws, which state the rights of the people and the powers of the government

contagions: diseases that are spread through close contact between people

executive: concerning the branch of government that includes the U.S. president, vice president, and cabinet

infrastructure: basic structures and facilities needed by society, such as buildings

judicial: concerning the part of government made up of the judges and justices who interpret laws and decide if they are constitutional

legislative: concerning the U.S. Congress, composed of the Senate and the House of Representatives

malaria: a serious disease that can be spread to humans from a certain type of mosquito

malnutrition: a serious health condition when a person's diet does not have enough nutrients

pathogens: viruses, bacteria, or other microorganisms that can cause disease

seasonal influenza: a respiratory infection, sometimes called the "flu," that is caused by influenza viruses that circulate around the world

surveillance: close observation or monitoring

UNICEF: a program of the United Nations that works to improve health, education, and nutrition of children around the world

vaccination: treatment of a disease by providing immunity against it

veto: an action by one branch of government to prevent another from doing something

INDEX

LIGHTBOX

SUPPLEMENTARY RESOURCES

Click on the plus icon found in the bottom left corner of each spread to open additional teacher resources.

- Download and print the book's quizzes and activities
- Access curriculum correlations
- Explore additional web applications that enhance the Lightbox experience

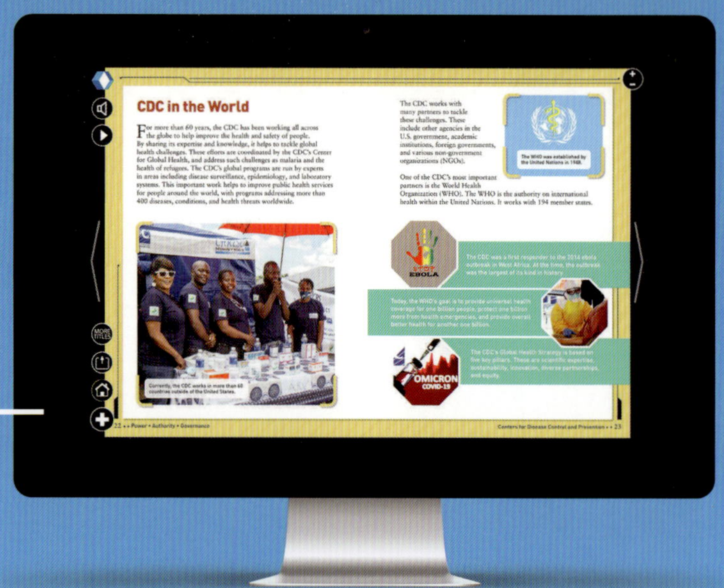

LIGHTBOX DIGITAL TITLES
Packed full of integrated media

VIDEOS

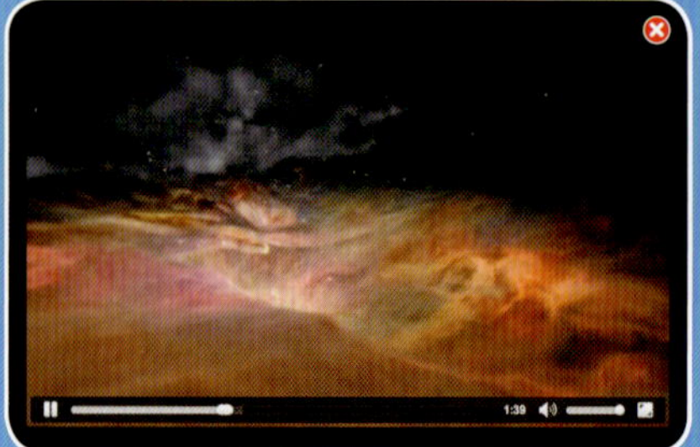

INTERACTIVE MAPS

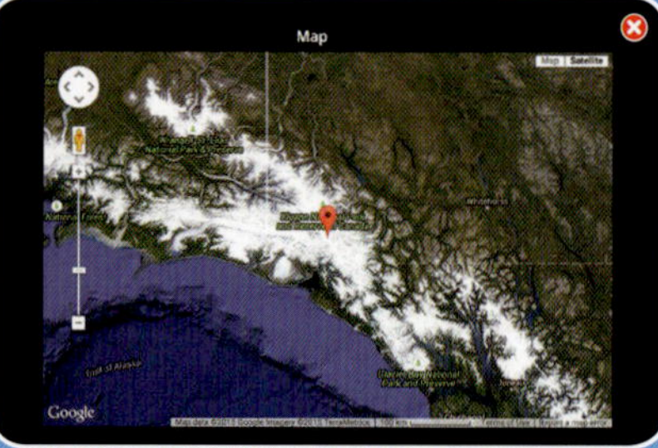

WEBLINKS

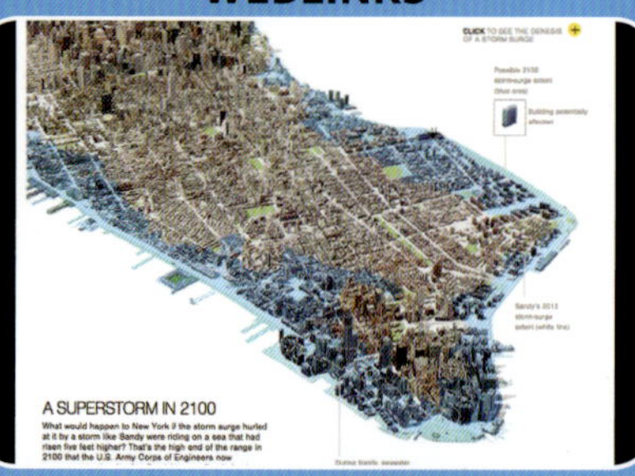

SLIDESHOWS

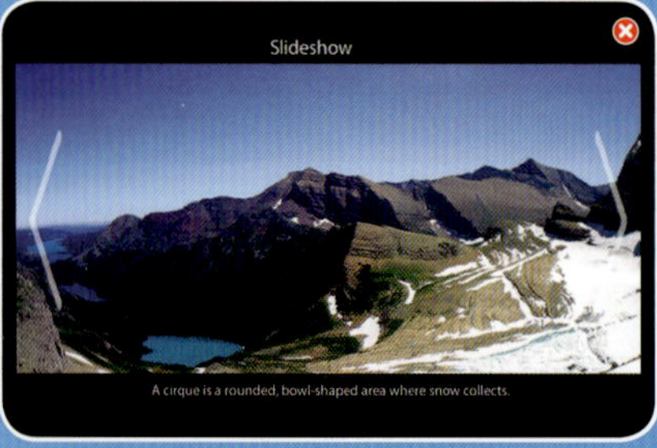

QUIZZES

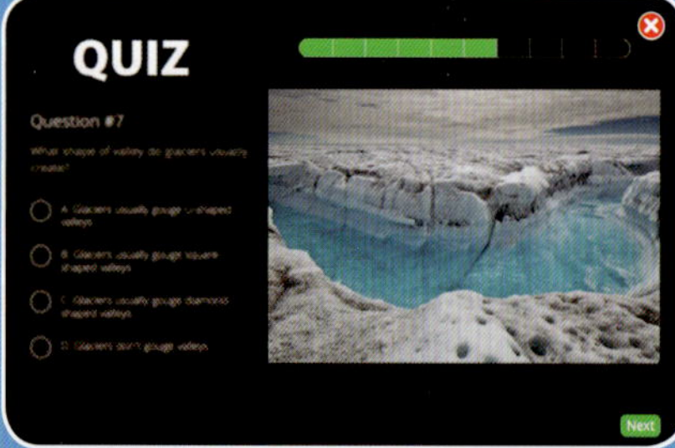

OPTIMIZED FOR

- ✓ TABLETS
- ✓ SMARTBOARDS
- ✓ COMPUTERS
- ✓ AND MUCH MORE!

Published by Lightbox Learning Inc.
276 5th Avenue, Suite 704 #917
New York, NY 10001
Website: www.openlightbox.com

Library of Congress Cataloging-in-Publication Data

Names: Beaucage, Adrienne, author.
Title: Centers for Disease Control and Prevention / Adrienne Beaucage.
Description: New York, NY : Smartbook Media Inc., [2022] | Series: Power, authority, and governance | Includes index. | Audience: Grades 4-6
Identifiers: LCCN 2021033726 (print) | LCCN 2021033727 (ebook) | ISBN 9781510558755 (library binding) | ISBN 9781510558762
Subjects: LCSH: Medicine, Preventive--Government policy--United States--Juvenile literature. | Centers for Disease Control and Prevention (U.S.)--Juvenile literature.
Classification: LCC RA445 .B389 2022 (print) | LCC RA445 (ebook) | DDC 614.4/4--dc23
LC record available at https://lccn.loc.gov/2021033726
LC ebook record available at https://lccn.loc.gov/2021033727

Printed in Guangzhou, China
1 2 3 4 5 6 7 8 9 0 27 26 25 24 23

012023
111121

Art Director: Terry Paulhus Project Coordinator: John Willis

Every reasonable effort has been made to trace ownership and to obtain permission to reprint copyright material. The publisher would be pleased to have any errors or omissions brought to its attention so that they may be corrected in subsequent printings.

The publisher acknowledges Alamy, Getty Images, Newscom, Shutterstock, and Wikimedia as the primary image suppliers for this title.